STRETCH MARKS

A Skincare Reference for Stretch Marks: A Comprehensive Guide to Diagnosis, Treatment, and Long-Term Skin Health

CHAD BRUNO

Table of Contents

Introductory

Strains, or stretch marks, are a frequent form of scarring that can emerge on the skin's surface. Discolorations can range in tone from pink or red to purple or brown, and can appear as elevated or depressed streaks or lines. Although stretch marks can appear anywhere on the body, they most frequently appear on the stomach, upper legs, hips, breasts, and arms.

Stretch marks are caused by the stretching of the skin beyond its usual boundaries. Several things might cause this stretching, including:

• Stretch marks can appear when the skin is unable to expand and contract at the same rate as the body, which can happen during puberty and pregnancy.

• Excessive weight gain can cause skin to stretch, especially if the weight is gained rapidly.

• Rapid muscular growth or bodybuilding can also cause stretch marks because the skin is stretched by the underlying muscles.

• **Use of Corticosteroids**: Topical or oral corticosteroid use over an extended period of time might decrease the skin's suppleness, increasing the risk of stretch marks.

• Puberty and other hormonal shifts, as well as some medical problems, might alter the skin's capacity to expand without tearing or scarring.

Stretch marks are a cosmetic issue for some people despite the fact that they are completely safe and offer no health hazards. Over time, they tend to diminish in color, becoming less prominent. The effectiveness of the many stretch mark creams, lotions, and treatments that claim to lessen their visibility varies.

These treatments may lessen the visibility of stretch marks, but they won't get rid of them entirely. Stretch marks can fade or even disappear completely with time with good treatment and hydration.

CHAPTER ONE
Stretch Marks: What We Know About Them

Striae distensae, or stretch marks, are a common skin ailment that are linked to alterations in the dermal connective tissue structure and composition. Stretch marks are related with a number of elements and scientific principles, but the specific mechanisms by which they arise are still a mystery.

1. Skin Elasticity and Collagen: The skin is formed of multiple layers, with the dermis being the layer responsible for preserving the skin's strength and elasticity. Two of the dermis' most important proteins are collagen and elastin. The skin's elasticity and resilience are made possible by elastin and collagen, respectively. Damage to these fibers can occur when the skin is stretched rapidly or for long periods of time.

2. Rupture of Connective Tissue: Rapid stretching of the skin (from pregnancy, weight growth, or other causes) can produce tears or disruptions in the collagen and elastin fibers in the dermis. This causes the skin to create fine scars that are visible as stretch marks.

3. Changes in hormone levels are another possible cause of stretch marks, along with hereditary factors. Hormonal shifts, for instance, may diminish the skin's elasticity during pregnancy. Some people may be more prone to getting stretch marks because of their genetic makeup.

4. Inflammatory Response: The early generation of stretch marks is related with an inflammatory response in the skin. The structure and pigmentation of the skin can change due to inflammation, making stretch marks more visible.

5. Microscopic alterations: Stretch marks are characterized by a region of reduced collagen and elastin content. Stretch marks may form in part because the dermal layer and the epidermal layer (the skin's outermost layer) both thin out.

6. Alterations to the blood vessels in the afflicted area can also have an effect on skin health by reducing blood flow to the skin.

Although various treatments have been suggested for stretch marks, including topical lotions, laser therapy, and microdermabrasion, unfortunately, none of them have been shown to be totally helpful for everyone. Although some of these treatments can help minimize the look of stretch marks by boosting collagen synthesis or smoothing the skin, they rarely result in a total disappearance of the scars.

Stretch mark formation is a multifaceted process, with visible and severe variations between individuals. While they may initially be red or purple in appearance, they frequently fade over time to a less visible white or silver shade. Maintaining a healthy skin care routine, including adequate hydration, can help diminish their look.

Stretch Marks and Pregnancy

Striae gravidarum, the medical term for stretch marks, are quite common during pregnancy. It's estimated that anywhere from 50 to 90 percent of pregnant women will develop stretch marks. Although these scars are most common on the stomach, they can also show up anywhere from the upper arms to the lower back. Here are some of the reasons why stretch marks are so common during pregnancy:

1. Pregnancy causes dramatic physical changes to the body, especially the belly, including rapid skin stretching. The skin's ability to adapt and expand without injury is exceeded by the rapid stretching of the skin caused by the uterus expanding as the baby grows.

2. Hormonal Variations: Stretch marks are more likely to appear during pregnancy because hormones like estrogen and relaxin reduce the skin's suppleness. Stretch marks may appear as a result of pregnancy's hormonal shifts and the higher blood volume.

3. Genetic Predisposition: Some women may be genetically inclined to acquiring stretch marks more easily. Stretch marks are hereditary, so if your mother or grandmother got them while pregnant, you can get them too.

4. Gaining weight is a common side effect of pregnancy because your body has to retain additional fat and fluids to nourish your growing baby. As the skin stretches to accommodate the additional weight, stretch marks may appear.

5. Women who have had numerous pregnancies, especially ones that were close together, are more likely to show signs of stretch marks.

While stretch marks are common during pregnancy and generally accepted as part of the process, many expectant mothers worry about how they will look. Some advice on how to deal with and lessen the appearance of stretch marks caused by pregnancy:

• Applying a moisturizing lotion or oil on a regular basis will help the skin retain its natural moisture and elasticity, both of which can lessen the appearance of stretch marks.

• By keeping your weight gain under control throughout pregnancy, you can lessen the likelihood of developing severe stretch marks.

• In order to keep your skin healthy and supple, be sure to drink lots of water.

• Massage using a light, emollient cream or oil has been shown to boost circulation and enhance skin condition.

• Care for your skin with moisturizers and treatments after having birth to aid in the gradual fading of stretch marks.

Even if stretch marks don't go away entirely, they usually lighten and fade with time, making them less of an eyesore. A dermatologist or other medical professional can

advise you on the best treatments
and products to use if you're self-
conscious about the look of your
stretch marks.

CHAPTER TWO
Growth Spurts and Puberty

Adolescents go through a time of rapid physical development and maturation known as puberty, which is closely tied to growth spurts. Growth in height and the appearance of secondary sexual features are just two of the many noticeable changes that occur to the body throughout puberty.

• Ages 8-13 for females and 9-14 for boys are common for the onset of puberty. The release of estrogen in females and testosterone in males triggers this process. Hormones like these tell the body it's time to begin sexual and physical development.

• Insulin-like growth factor 1 (IGF-1) and growth hormone (GH) are two of the main growth hormones that are secreted throughout puberty. These hormones cause the epiphyseal plates (the ends of long bones) to expand, resulting in longer bones.

• Midway through puberty is often when a person has the greatest growth spurt. This growth spurt typically begins in girls around the age of 10 and in boys around the age of 12, though there is some variation. Different people develop at different rates.

• The lengthening of long bones such as the arms, legs, and spine during the growth spurt is a major factor in the overall rise in stature. Skeletal maturity, which normally occurs in one's late teens or early twenties, causes the growth plates to fuse together and seal.

• Secondary sexual features, such as breast development in girls and a deeper voice in boys, appear throughout puberty, coinciding with the teenage growth spurt. Hormonal fluctuations are the primary cause of this variability.

• Redistribution of Body Fat: As puberty advances, there are shifts in where fat is stored in the body, where muscle grows, and what form the body takes. While boys gain muscle mass and decrease body fat, girls gain width at the hips and subcutaneous fat.

• Along with the physical, puberty is a time of significant emotional and psychological development. As they face the obstacles of becoming an adult, adolescents often go through a period of emotional, identity, and social upheaval.

It's worth noting that each person experiences puberty and subsequent growth spurts at their own unique timetable and at their own unique rate. How quickly and how much a person grows during this time can be affected by factors like genetics, nutrition, general health, and environmental influences.

When a person's growth plates fuse together, they often cease becoming taller. The complete puberty process, including growth spurts, can take many years; by the time teenagers reach full physical and sexual maturity, the body has stabilized.

Stretch Marks and Weight Gain

Changes in body weight, whether from rapid weight gain or decrease, can affect the formation and visibility of stretch marks. Stretch marks form when the skin is stretched rapidly, which can happen as a result of pregnancy or rapid weight gain or loss. Here's how the correlation between weight swings and stretch marks works:

1. **Weight Gain:** When a person gains a substantial amount of

weight in a very short period, the skin may not be able to adjust to the increased size quickly enough. Stretch marks are commonly seen on the breasts, stomach, thighs, and hips because of the rapid stretching of the skin during pregnancy. Stretch marks arise when the skin's collagen and elastin fibers, which give it strength and suppleness, are destroyed.

2. Pregnancy: The development of the fetus and shifts in the body's fluid balance usually lead to a substantial increase in weight during pregnancy. Stretch marks may appear on the abdomen when the skin stretches to accommodate the growing baby. And because of the hormonal shifts that occur during pregnancy, your skin may be less elastic and more prone to stretch marks.

3. Although weight increase is more commonly associated with the appearance of stretch marks, rapid weight loss can also play a role. This is because the skin may take some time to go back to its pre-stretched state after rapid weight loss. Although stretch marks may not be as widespread in cases of weight loss as they are in cases of weight gain, they can nonetheless emerge as a result of the loose skin.

It's worth noting that everyone's stretch mark experience is unique. There may be a hereditary predisposition for stretch marks, or some people may simply have skin that is more resistant to stretching than others. Although stretch marks may be unsightly, they are not harmful in any other way.

Stretch marks caused by weight changes can be treated and concealed by:

• Hydrate Your Skin Consistently Skin elasticity and appearance can be enhanced by regular moisturization.

• Keep Your Weight Even: Stretch marks are less likely to appear if your weight does not fluctuate too much or too quickly.

• Laser therapy and topical treatments may help reduce the visibility of existing stretch marks; discuss these options with your dermatologist.

• Even without treatment, stretch marks tend to diminish and become less apparent with time.

There may not be a foolproof method to prevent stretch marks, but these techniques can help minimize their visibility over time.

CHAPTER THREE
Procedures and Treatments in Medicine

The term "medical treatment" refers to a broad category of diagnostic and therapeutic techniques used to address a wide range of health issues. Doctors, surgeons, nurses, and other medical specialists are the usual people who administer these treatments and procedures. Some broad classifications of medical interventions include:

1. Methods of Diagnosis:

• X-rays, CT scans, MRI, ultrasound, and PET scans are all examples of medical imaging techniques used to create an image of the body's interior for the purposes of diagnosis and follow-up care.

Biopsies are used to detect cancer and other disorders by analyzing samples of tissue from the body.

Infections, diabetes, and autoimmune illnesses can all be detected with a simple blood test.

2. Operative Techniques:

- **General Surgery:** Includes treatments include appendectomies, gallbladder removal, and hernia repair.

• Cardiac Surgery entails operations on the heart, including as angioplasty and valve replacement.

Surgery performed on the musculoskeletal system, such as joint replacements, fracture repairs, and spinal procedures.

Brain and nervous system operations, such as tumor removal and spinal treatments, are under the umbrella of neurosurgery.

3. Therapeutic Interventions:

• Medication refers to the use of pharmaceuticals for the purpose of treating, preventing, or managing illness. Medicines can be taken orally, applied topically, or injected.

Common cancer treatments include chemotherapy and radiation therapy, both of which work by killing cancer cells.

Immunotherapy: a method of treating cancer and other diseases by stimulating the immune system.

• Antibiotic Treatment: Used for Infections Caused by Bacteria.

4. Methods with a Small Incision:

• The term "endoscopy" refers to the use of a flexible tube equipped with a camera to inspect and treat inside body parts.

- Laparoscopy is a minimally invasive surgical method used for appendectomies and gallbladder removals that is conducted through small incisions.

Minimally invasive procedures like angioplasty and embolization are examples of what are known as "interventional radiology," which uses image guidance to perform the procedures.

5. Therapies for Recovery

• Restoring mobility and strength after an injury is made possible by physical therapists.

• The goal of occupational therapy is to help patients become more independent in their daily lives by teaching them new skills and retraining them in old ones.

Individuals with speech and language impairments, such as stuttering or aphasia, can benefit from speech therapy.

6. Complementary and alternative medicine:

• Acupuncture is a pain-relieving and health-enhancing practice that makes use of the insertion of very thin needles into precise anatomical locations all over the body.

Chiropractic treatment for musculoskeletal disorders focuses on spinal manipulation and adjustments.

• **Herbal Medicine:** The use of plant-based therapies for various health conditions.

7. Therapies for Mental Illness:

• Psychotherapy entails talking sessions with a licensed therapist to work through emotional and mental difficulties.

Prescribed to treat mental health disorders such as depression, anxiety, and bipolar disorder.

8. In the field of dentistry, services range from the simple to the sophisticated, including everything from checkups and cleanings to root canals and braces.

9. Rehabilitation, prosthetic fittings, and modifications to assistive technology are all examples of physical and occupational operations.

10. Aesthetic procedures are generally carried out by plastic surgeons and dermatologists, and include things like Botox injections, facelifts, and breast augmentation.

The diagnosis, severity, and other considerations all have a role in determining the course of treatment or operation that is advised. In order to determine the best course of action to take for their health, patients should speak with their healthcare providers about their concerns, preferences, and options.

Home Treatments and Organic Medicines

Health, minor discomforts, and emotional support can all benefit from using natural treatments and home care techniques. These cures and practices often entail the use of natural products and basic approaches. They may not be able to substitute conventional medical care for severe disorders, but they can help with many everyday health issues. Here are some home care techniques and natural cures for common health problems:

1. Fevers and Colds:

• Water, herbal teas, and broths, along with plenty of other fluids, can help alleviate symptoms and prevent dehydration.

If you have a sore throat or a cough, try a blend of honey and lemon.

2. Headaches:

• If you have a headache, try rubbing some diluted peppermint oil on your temples.

Tea made from ginger root has been shown to alleviate headache pain.

3. Acid Reflux / Indigestion:

- **Ginger:** Chewing ginger or drinking ginger tea might ease stomach discomfort.

A mixture of a little baking soda and water will help ease heartburn temporarily.

4. Diarrhea and vomiting:

- If you're feeling queasy, try some ginger candies, ginger tea, or ginger chews.

Peppermint can help settle an upset stomach when consumed in the form of peppermint tea or peppermint candies.

5. Injuries of a Minimal Nature:

• Honey contains antimicrobial properties and helps speed the recovery of small cuts and scrapes.

The gel extracted from the aloe vera plant can be used to treat small burns and other skin irritations, and it also has a calming effect.

6. Disorders of the Skin:

• Itching and irritation caused by skin diseases like eczema can be soothed with an oatmeal bath.

Acne and fungus-related skin problems may respond favorably to diluted tea tree oil.

7. Insomnia:

• Chamomile Tea: Chamomile tea is a natural sleep aid that can encourage calm.

• **Lavender**: Diffusing or applying lavender oil to the skin might help relieve stress.

8. Difficulty Moving:

• Sore muscles can be soothed and inflammation quelled with the aid of an Epsom salt bath.

Applying arnica gel directly to the skin can help alleviate muscle pain.

9. Congestion:

• Nasal congestion and sore throats can be alleviated by inhaling steam from a bowl of hot water.

The nasal passages can be cleansed with a saline solution rinse.

10. Anxiety and Stress:

• Stress and anxiety can be better handled by doing deep breathing techniques.

Regular practice of meditation and yoga has been shown to improve both physical and mental health.

While many people have found success with natural cures and self-care techniques like these, it's important to keep in mind that they may not be the best option for everyone. Consult your doctor before utilizing natural remedies if you have a medical problem, are taking drugs, or are worried about your health. Furthermore, it is often vital to seek medical attention from a trained specialist when dealing with serious or persistent health difficulties.

CHAPTER FOUR
Marks of Male Puberty

Stretch marks, commonly known as striae, can afflict both men and women. Stretch marks are more common in women, especially during pregnancy, although males can get them for a number of different reasons. The most common causes of stretch marks in men are as follows:

• Adolescent growth spurts are not limited to females; males can experience them as well. Stretch marks are common among athletes because of the rapid gain in height and muscle mass, especially on the thighs, buttocks, and lower back.

• Obesity and excessive weight gain: The skin's elastic properties are exceeded when the body's fat stores are expanded beyond their normal range of motion. Stretch marks are a common side effect of pregnancy, especially on the stomach, hips, and upper arms.

• Muscle can be developed rapidly with bodybuilding and weightlifting workouts. Stretch marks are scars that occur on the skin, most commonly on the shoulders, upper arms, and thighs, as a result of rapid muscle growth and other physical changes.

• Muscle growth is accelerated by the use of anabolic steroids, which are sometimes used to improve sports performance and in the context of bodybuilding. Due to the skin's inability to accommodate this expansion, stretch marks may appear.

• Overproduction of the hormone cortisol is at the root of Cushing's syndrome, a medical disorder that causes significant weight gain, muscle weakness, and skin abnormalities, including the appearance of stretch marks.

• Some people may have a higher predisposition to stretch marks due to their genes. You could be more likely to get stretch marks if either of your parents or other close relatives had them.

Stretch marks on men can be any color, but most commonly they are pink, red, purple, or brown. They eventually turn a silvery white and become less apparent as time passes. Some men may worry about how they look, despite the fact that they offer no health risk.

The following methods may be tried in order to control and lessen the visibility of stretch marks in males:

- Creams and oils available for purchase without a prescription have been shown to reduce the visibility of stretch marks. Ingredients like retinoids, hyaluronic acid, and vitamin E might be present in these goods.

- This cosmetic technique, known as microneedling, makes use of a device with extremely thin needles in order to improve the skin's texture and stimulate collagen synthesis.

- Some types of laser therapy are effective in reducing the visibility of stretch marks.

- Tanning: Tanning can help conceal stretch marks by making them stand out less against the darker skin. However, safety measures must be taken to prevent overexposure to the sun and subsequent skin damage.

If a man is worried about stretch marks, he should talk to a doctor or dermatologist to get advice on the best treatments and products for his situation.

Staying Stretch Mark-Free

It may not always be feasible to avoid getting stretch marks, but there are things you can do to lessen their chance and the impact they have on your body. Here are some suggestions for avoiding unsightly stretch marks:

- Stretch marks are a common result of rapid weight gain or decrease; therefore it's important to keep your weight stable. Try to keep your weight where it should be by eating healthily and exercising frequently. Stretch marks are less likely to appear during a slow, steady weight gain or loss.

- **Stay moisturized:** Drinking enough of water helps keep your skin moisturized and retains its suppleness. Skin that is well moisturized is less likely to show signs of stretching.

• Applying a high-quality moisturizer on a regular basis will help prevent stretch marks, especially in vulnerable areas like the stomach, thighs, and buttocks. The flexibility of your skin can be enhanced by using a moisturizer with hyaluronic acid, cocoa butter, or shea butter.

• A healthy diet that's rich in vitamins and minerals can help your skin look and feel its best. Vitamins A, C, and E, as well as zinc and silica, should be prioritized in your diet. Having healthy skin requires these nutrients.

• Foods High in Collagen-Supporting Nutrients Foods high in collagen-supporting nutrients can aid in maintaining skin suppleness. Bone broth, seafood, and lean proteins are all examples.

• For some, taking dietary supplements like vitamin E or fish oil can have a positive impact on skin quality. Before starting any new supplement regimen, talk to your doctor.

• When lifting weights or engaging in bodybuilding, it's preferable to build muscle slowly rather than quickly to avoid the onset of stretch marks.

• Consult your doctor about laser therapy and other options to reduce the likelihood of getting stretch marks before undergoing surgery or a major weight reduction.

• **Pregnancy**: Moisturizers should be applied to the belly and breasts on a daily basis, and expectant moms should maintain a healthy weight.

• Steroids should be avoided if at all possible; those who are already using them should use caution when trying to prevent stretch marks.

• Avoid getting too much sun, as it can harm the skin's suppleness and make stretch marks more likely to appear.

• Keep in mind that your genetic makeup can also affect your susceptibility to getting stretch marks. You can get stretch marks if there's a history of them in your family.

However, it's crucial to remember that these treatments may not be 100% effective because other factors, like genetics and life circumstances, can play a part in whether or not you end up with stretch marks. Additionally, if you have existing stretch marks, there are many treatments, including topical lotions, laser therapy, and microdermabrasion, that can help improve their look. A dermatologist or other healthcare professional can give you individualized recommendations and treatment plans.

Conclusion

Rapid weight gain or loss, hormonal shifts, pregnancy, and even heredity can all contribute to the development of stretch marks, a common skin issue. They don't hurt your health and aren't dangerous, but many people are self-conscious about how they look. These skin discolorations typically appear as pink, crimson, or purple streaks at first, but over time they lighten to a silvery-white tint.

Maintaining a healthy lifestyle, including progressive weight management, enough hydration, and a balanced diet, is essential for managing and preventing stretch marks. Supporting skin health and lowering the likelihood of stretch marks can also be accomplished by using moisturizers and collagen-boosting substances. Although it may not always be practicable, these methods can help reduce the severity and duration of stretch marks.

Topical lotions, laser therapy, and other medical interventions are available for persons with existing stretch marks or who are concerned about their appearance. For specific guidance and treatment choices, it's best to speak with a healthcare physician or dermatologist.

Stretch marks are a normal part of the aging process, and they in no way reflect on a person's value or attractiveness. They're totally natural and common, and many people find ways to celebrate their bodies despite having a few flaws here and there.

THE END